Contemporary Issues

Leading Girls to Mathematics, Science, and Technology

Into the World of Today and Tomorrow

Girl Scouts of the U.S.A.
420 Fifth Avenue
New York, N.Y. 10018-2702

GIRL SCOUTS OF THE U.S.A.®

Betty F. Pilsbury, *President*
Frances Hesselbein, *National Executive Director*

Inquiries related to *Contemporary Issues: Into the World of Today and Tomorrow* should be directed to Membership and Program, Girl Scouts of the U.S.A., 420 Fifth Avenue, New York, N.Y. 10018-2702.

Author: Sharon Woods Hussey

Contributors: Candace White Ciraco
Margaret Andrews

Editor: Susan Eno

This publication was produced with the assistance of a grant from The Weyerhaeuser Company Foundation.

First Impression 1987
Printed in the United States of America
10 9 8 7 6
ISBN 0-88441-463-9

Contents

The Girl Scout Contemporary Issues Series

Tune In to Well-Being, Say No to Drugs: Substance Abuse

Staying Safe: Preventing Child Abuse

Girls Are Great: Growing Up Female

Into the World of Today and Tomorrow: Leading Girls to Mathematics, Science, and Technology

Reaching Out: Preventing Youth Suicide

Caring and Coping: Facing Family Crises

Decisions for Your Life: Preventing Teenage Pregnancy

Earth Matters: A Challenge for Environmental Action

Valuing Differences: Pluralism

Right to Read: Literacy

Introduction

As society hurtles toward the twenty-first century, one trend stands out clearly: The fabric of our lives continues to be progressively interwoven with the sciences. Scientific advances affect everything from the very beginnings of life to explorations into the furthest reaches of the universe. Developments in the sciences reflect human strivings to comprehend and improve every aspect of life so that everyone will live in a better future. Girls today need support and encouragement to become active participants in the scientific, mathematical, and technological work that will shape their future.

Girls and women live in a world that offers greater choices and more opportunities than ever before. However, despite these expanded options, some critical choices are being ignored—choices to venture into courses of study and employment in mathematics and science. Instead, many girls opt for career paths that avoid these subjects. As a result, they ultimately limit their understanding, enjoyment, and employment in these fields and related technologies. They may also fail to achieve sufficient mathematical and scientific understanding to become fully knowledgeable citizens.

Although we are a society growing increasingly dependent on mathematics, the sciences, and resultant technologies, women are dramatically underrepresented in these fields at every level. (This is also true for Blacks, Hispanics, American Indians, and people with disabilities.) In spite of great strides in breaking down the barriers of the past, the evidence shows that girls are not entering the fields of mathematics and science in numbers comparable to boys.

This scenario is further complicated by growing concern that the United States as a whole seriously lags behind other countries around the world in the study of mathematics and science.

Why Encourage Girls to Pursue Studies in Mathematics and the Sciences?

It has been said that to wonder is to begin to understand. Girl Scouting can help girls see that science and mathematics are wonderful.

It is critical to help girls view science- and math-related career choices as valid and desirable. Not only does lack of involvement deny them the right to shape their future, it carries economic consequences as well. Employment opportunities in positions in new technological fields are projected to grow at faster rates than opportunities in many current fields. Research shows that serious deficiencies in mathematics and science can have considerable impact on one's earning power and upward mobility on the career ladder. In short, opportunities to progress along a career path can be seriously limited without sufficient background in mathematics and science.

Many characterize present twentieth-century life as the information age. A driving force in today's society is the creation, production, and distribution of information. And, it is the application of discoveries in mathematics and science that makes information technologies possible.

Although none of the following examples appear particularly unusual today, past generations would have been utterly amazed by the information technology that makes it possible to:

- Complete banking transactions with plastic cards and display terminals.
- See live events from all around the world.
- Have supermarket cash registers automatically scan the descriptions and prices of groceries.
- Record and instantly play back a video of a family party or event.
- Take pictures of the surfaces of Mars, Jupiter, and other planets.

Girls, Women, Science—The Facts Show the Need for Change

- Women make up 52 percent of the work force but only 7 percent of the engineers.[1]

- Elementary schools spend an average of only 15 minutes a day on science education, and that is usually spent reading textbooks rather than in hands-on activities.

The number of students earning science and engineering doctorates in the U.S. has steadily decreased and is now at its lowest level since 1968.

Both statements made by Senator Edward Kennedy as he introduced legislation on April 19, 1990, for the Mathematics, Science and Engineering Bill (S.2114).

- Women scientists and engineers represented about 13 percent of the science and engineering work force in 1986, up from 11 percent in 1980.[2]

- During the elementary and middle-school years, female students are less likely to have the kind of extracurricular experiences that foster an interest in science or engineering. Many studies also indicate that, although girls' grades are similar to or better than boys', teachers tend to hold lower expectations for girls in science and mathematics.[3]

- Males make up 77 percent of this country's computer science majors, 77 percent of its working computer analysts, and 93 percent of its home computer users, according to the 1984 Scientific Manpower Commission survey.[4]

- In 1985, women earned 27 percent of medical degrees and 36 percent of law degrees.[5]

- Seventeen percent of the high technology professionals in Silicon Valley are women.[6]

- Junior and senior high schools nationwide report that most of the students who use computers in their free time are boys.[7]

Getting Started

Just a few quick definitions before starting. The terms "science," "mathematics," and "technology" are being used here in their broadest senses. In very simple terms, science is the pursuit of the answers to the what, why, and how of life and the universe. The object of scientific study may vary, but there is always a desire and effort to see, know, understand, and explain. Mathematics is the study of numbers and shapes, their forms and relationships. Technology puts the discoveries of mathematics and science—those answers to how, what, and why—into action.

What resources do you need to help girls explore these fields? Contrary to popularly held misconceptions, you don't need fancy, expensive, or hard-to-find equipment. You don't need a doctoral degree or the I.Q. of a genius. What do you need?

- A sense of wonder and curiosity about everything and anything.

- The desire to explore and the ability to remain undaunted by unexpected changes. Explorations, experiments, and discoveries rarely go exactly as planned, and many important discoveries come from the unexpected.

- An open mind and a willingness to venture into something new.

- The conviction that girls must be encouraged in these fields and that Girl Scouting can make a difference.

Why Do Many Girls Avoid Mathematics, Science, and Technology?

There is no conclusive evidence to prove that sex-related differences in mathematics or science achievement stem from genetic, hormonal, or physiological differences. The entire body of evidence indicates that the reasons why females have historically lagged behind males are quite

[1]Stronch, David R., "Problems of Teaching Science to Girls," *Contemporary Education,* Vol. LX, No. 4 (Terre Haute, Ind.: Indiana State University, 1989), pp. 223–225.
[2]National Science Board, *Science and Engineering Indicators—1989* (Washington, D.C.: U.S. Government Printing Office, 1989).
[3]Matyas, Marsha Lakes, and June Burton Combs, *Girl Scouts, Science and Mathematics: Linkages for the Future* (Washington, D.C.: American Association for the Advancement of Science, 1989).
[4]"Closing the Gender Gap," *Teaching and Computers,* Vol. 4, Issue 7 (New York, N.Y.: Scholastic Inc., 1987), p. 8.
[5]Kreinberg, Nancy, "Women and Mathematics: An Update," *California Women.* Issue 3 (Sacramento, Calif.: California Commission on the Status of Women, 1986), p. 5.
[6]Gilliland, Kay, "EQUALS in Computer Technology," *The Computing Teacher* (1984).

[7]Sanders, Jo, *Do Your Female Students Say "No Thanks" to the Computer?* (New York, N.Y.: Women's Action Alliance, 1987).

complex. Educational and social influences play a major role.

Educational Influences

The encouraging fact is that numerous studies indicate girls start out ahead of boys in school in practically all areas, including speaking, reading, and counting. By age thirteen, consistent sex-related differences emerge on standardized texts. Although girls often still receive better classroom grades, scores for girls in mathematics and science on standardized achievement tests lag behind those of boys. In the classroom, girls are often rewarded for being quiet and compliant. The reinforcement of these characteristics can hinder the development of self-reliance and independence.

Recent studies indicate that girls are more likely to be "invisible" members of classrooms—receiving fewer teacher contacts and less instruction in how to do things for themselves. For example, by age nine, girls have fewer opportunities to work with science materials, observe natural phenomena, conduct experiments, or participate in extracurricular science activities. By the junior/senior high school years, girls are already dismissing careers requiring higher-level mathematics.

Girl Scouting can be a powerful force in counteracting some of these trends. In the accepting environment of a Girl Scout group, led by an encouraging leader, girls can exercise their self-reliance and put their skills and talents into action. The opportunity for Daisy, Brownie, and Junior Girl Scout leaders to make a difference is particularly significant. Girls at these age levels certainly have the capabilities, and most have not yet yielded to the pressures and influences that cause girls to avoid mathematics and science.

Schools may be part of the problem. A survey by the American Psychological Association revealed that many school counselors continue to foster traditional sex roles when counseling female students. And unfortunately, many educators do not strongly encourage girls to study higher mathematics and the sciences. These lowered expectations for girls affect self-esteem and self-confidence. Girls begin to believe they can not do better and often don't.

Textbooks and curriculum materials with sexist biases are another problem. Studies have shown that examples and illustrations—especially in math and science texts—are directed primarily toward boys. Lack of female role models in texts is another problem. Often, pictures in math books portray more males than females. One method of eliminating such biases often creates another. For some texts the solution has been not to depict people of either sex. This, however, does nothing to counteract a girl's belief that science or math is not for her.

Here again, the message for Girl Scout leaders is that you can make a difference. One way is to help girls explore World of Today and Tomorrow activities in the Girl Scout resources. When mathematical and scientific courses of study are not linked with real-life situations, too often girls are left wondering, "How does this connect to my life?" or "How will I ever use this?" The Girl Scout materials are designed specifically for girls and can enable them to explore their own world.

Girls may have the misperception that mathematics and science involve learning one acceptable method that will yield only one right answer. Place value on experimentation and try different approaches. Encourage girls to guess and make intuitive attempts at problem-solving. Early on, many students perceive that asking questions translates into looking dumb; as a consequence, natural curiosity may be stifled and confusion left unresolved. This is especially a problem for girls who tend to associate making mistakes with moral judgments. You can help girls to enjoy finding answers and see that everyone has questions.

Another problem is that many females are not becoming sufficiently computer literate. In many academic programming courses around the country, boys outnumber girls by as many as two to one. Evidence shows that this discrepancy is a result of psychological barriers and patterns of subtle discrimination rather than differences in abilities. For example, some computer software and computer games have designs that appeal more to boys than to girls.

The very encouraging news comes from a National Science Foundation survey that found a positive correlation between early learning experiences and later achievement in mathematics and science. When girls are provided with a wide variety of experiences that expose them to math and science, they will be far less likely to avoid these subjects in the future. That means that Girl Scouting can take a lead role in providing those necessary early positive experiences that can make a difference in girls' lives.

Social Influences

From infancy through early childhood, girls receive subtle and not so subtle messages that mathematics and science are male domains. Although changes are occurring, career-oriented toys such as building blocks, erector sets, science and doctors' kits have been directed toward boys. The problem is further compounded by a lack of visible role models. By secondary school there is an overall decrease in female teachers and there is an even more noticeable lack of females instructing in math and science courses of study. Further, there are simply not enough women dentists, engineers, physicists, and mathematicians for young girls to identify with. It is especially important for minority youths to see others from a similar cultural background who are actively engaged in mathematical or scientific pursuits.

The phenomenon known as "learned helplessness" also plays a role. All too often we hear females attribute a shortcoming or failure to inability—they take an "I can't do it" attitude. This becomes a self-fulfilling prophecy: As girls convince themselves that they cannot do things, this indeed comes to be true. Likewise, many females attribute their successes to "being lucky" instead of taking credit for the ability and effort that were most likely responsible. This is further complicated by a tendency—especially displayed by bright girls—to be perfectionistic while devaluing what they do well.

Interestingly, some research suggests that success is not always a comfortable notion. Studies show that some females fear that their femininity might be compromised if they are too capable, especially should they seriously pursue male-dominated careers such as those in mathematics and science. There is also evidence that at the college level females avoid math and science majors because they fail to envision how such a career would successfully combine with marriage and family.

Overcoming Fears

Self-reliance, competence, success—all have been encouraged by Girl Scouting since its very beginning. Juliette Low urged girls to be all that they could. This is still the case today. Without the right support and encouragement, many girls begin to believe that they simply don't have what it takes to successfully pursue courses of study in mathematics and science. Some feel anxiety or even panic when confronted with these subjects. A self-defeating cycle of avoidance and failure often occurs. Many girls experience bouts of loss of self-esteem. Although these reactions may sound extreme, they are very real to the persons experiencing them. The end effect is a large body of people—mostly females—who feel discouraged and withdrawn, and are math and science disabled. This pattern is especially dysfunctional for Black, Hispanic, and American Indian females, who have an extra cultural bias to deal with. But the pattern can be altered: Girl Scout leaders have the perfect opportunity to lead girls into the world of today and tomorrow.

Specific Tips for Girl Scout Leaders

Provide positive reinforcement:

■ Help girls to have a sense of well-being and experience success in an activity. This makes it much more likely that they will continue their involvement.

■ Be sure to praise the girls for their efforts, since many girls tend to evaluate themselves on the basis of how a "significant other" (i.e., parent, teacher, troop leader, peer) perceives them.

■ Give active encouragement to the girls. The absence of any positive comment or action is often construed by girls to be a negative rather than neutral response.

■ Give special attention to underachieving girls, who need encouragement and support from a caring adult partner.

■ Encourage and model values of perseverance and persistence. Having the ability to persist in the face of conflict or failure is directly related to a positive self-concept.

■ Encourage girls to take risks, to trust their intuition, and to avoid self-defeating talk. Don't fall into the trap of sympathizing by saying, "That's O.K., I didn't like math or science either."

■ Develop an active partnership with the girls, especially in decision-making. Encourage problem-solving skills—ask how and why questions.

■ Help the girls to explore their own feelings and attitudes. You might discuss how they feel about mathematics and science, exactly what they like or dislike, and how the study of these fields could be made better.

■ Develop projects that allow for cooperative group work. Research demonstrates that females tend to prefer a collaborative work style.

■ Create competitive situations that are as nonthreatening as possible.

Encourage the development of mathematical and scientific skills:

■ Build models, take measurements, construct things.

■ Encourage girls to play with games and puzzles. Jigsaw puzzles and strategy games strengthen logical thinking, problem-solving skills, and visual-spatial skills.

■ Play counting games.

Help make mathematics/science study more interesting, attractive, and relevant:

■ Help girls to see how mathematics and science can be part of the solution for human, social, environmental, and ecological concerns.

■ Help girls find successful female role models.

■ Be tuned in to community-based organizations, museums, universities, nature centers, etc., that can be helpful in providing resources and adult role models.

■ Impart an awareness of the many career opportunities available to girls through math- and science-based curriculum study.

■ Find activities involving science and mathematics in all the Girl Scout worlds of interest.

■ Combine science and math with nonscience and math activities. Have a "camp-in" in a science museum. Sing a counting song.

Be an advocate:

■ Expect the best from every girl.

■ Increase your own personal knowledge of mathematics, science, and technology. (See the Resources section in this book for ideas.)

■ Be sensitive to signs of math or science anxiety/avoidance in yourself and in individual girls.

■ Develop links with school personnel, especially counselors, to help you plan activities.

■ Raise the awareness of others. Help them appreciate the need to encourage girls in these fields.

■ Be confident of your own ability to explore new areas.

■ Be aware of sex-role stereotyping in books and other resources.

Suggested Troop/Group Activities for Exploring Mathematics, Science, and Technology

The same reasons that ultimately cause girls to withdraw from science- and math-related courses of study in school and later in career paths are also at work with respect to Girl Scout program. Mathematics and science have been, since the very beginning of Girl Scouting, the foundation of many enjoyable activities. However, the evidence shows that girls and leaders may be more reluctant to attempt activities in the World of Today and Tomorrow than activities from the other worlds of interest.

The following activity suggestions are designed to help girls discover that explorations in mathematics, science, and technology can be fun and easy. The activity lists are not categorized by Girl Scout age level but instead by type of activity. They do not attempt to turn Girl Scout leaders into instant scientists, nor do they duplicate any of the multitude of activities already in the program resources. Instead, the activities help communicate the basic message that science, mathematics, and technology are a constant part of life today, in both obvious and not so obvious ways, and that exploring these fields is fun and exciting. Most of the activities are easily adaptable to each program age level. Some activities may be more appropriate for younger or for older girls, and in some instances specific tips for a particular age level are given. It is recommended that Girl Scout groups explore at least one activity in each section.

Be sure to refer to the Resources section of this booklet. There you will find listings of relevant organizations, museums, science centers, magazines, books, and other publications that can help science, mathematics, and technology to come alive for your Girl Scouts.

Creative, Fun Explorations

1. Select at least five new activities to try from the Program Links in this booklet (pages 15–16).

2. Earn a new recognition in the World of Today and Tomorrow.

3. Build something that meets a challenge.

- A stack of blocks higher than the tallest girl
- A trail that won't wash away in the rain
- A sand castle with three openings
- A place to store group projects
- Design your own challenging project

4. Include puzzle solving, strategy games, riddle contests, or similar problem-solving activities in at least four meetings.

5. Watch one of the special television series that focus on mathematics or science. *Nova, Square One, 3-2-1 Contact, Nature, The Know Zone, Innovation*, and National Geographic specials are just some examples. (Check local TV listings for time and channel.) After viewing a show, discuss the roles of scientists or mathematicians and what was learned.

6. Try at least five of the activities in the "Computers and You" and "Girls + Math = Fun" insert in this booklet.

7. Put on a science/math magic show. Some ideas to consider are optical illusions, number games, magic squares, or tricks that put chemistry, biology, physics, or some other science into action.

8. Make a toy that uses science or math. Know what makes it work and why.

9. Visit and explore at least one of the following:

- Science museum
- Nature center
- Aquarium
- Planetarium
- Natural history museum
- Zoo

If you are not able to visit one of the above, see if there are any traveling exhibits coming to your area. Or, start your own discovery room or activities center that allows for hands-on experiences.

10. Try some kitchen chemistry experiments. There's a lot you can do with everyday cooking ingredients.

1. For one day, keep track of all the technologies upon which you depend. Compare your day to what it may have been like 100 years ago, and imagine what it could be like 100 years in the future.

2. Try one or more of the following:

- Have someone show you the main parts of a car engine.
- Take apart a discarded appliance.
- Help someone fix an appliance.
- Operate a computer.

3. Find out how at least one of the following has changed because of new technology.

- Medical diagnoses and treatments
- Transportation
- Help for people with disabilities
- Means of communication
- Banking
- Agriculture and food processing
- ? ? any area that interests you

4. Start a file on mathematics, science, and technology in the news, including clippings from both newspapers and magazines. Find a way to share the file with others.

5. In the quest for answers and the development of technology based on scientific discoveries, many groups may be affected and people are often faced with new moral and ethical dilemmas. Find out about and discuss one or more of the following issues.

- Computer fraud
- Acid rain
- Gene splicing
- Protection of endangered species
- Videocassette and audiotape piracy
- Medical experiments with animals
- The possibility of life elsewhere in the universe
- In vitro fertilization
- Nuclear waste disposal
- Use of pesticides
- Changes in the ozone layer of the atmosphere

6. Many of the world's problems have their greatest impact on women. Find out about and discover how science and technology may offer solutions to:

- Illiteracy. The number of females who cannot read is greater than the number of males.
- Water supplies. In many areas there is not an adequate supply of safe, clean water. The problem is especially great in third-world countries.
- Old age. In most cultures women outlive men, and the care of the aged is usually the responsibility of women.
- Malnutrition. Millions of people around the world, including many in the United States, are not adequately nourished. Many millions die from starvation and millions more suffer from malnutrition.
- Immunization and disease. Millions of children around the world still die from diseases that can be prevented or cured through proper health practices and medical care.

7. Imagine some technological breakthroughs that might be possible 50 years from now. Discuss the benefits and possible problems that might come about with these advances. Write a science fiction story or put on a play that incorporates these technological advances into the plot.

8. With a group of older girls, discuss two or more of the following facts, considering possible reasons and potential impact.

Did You Know?

- The number of women in the labor force has tripled in the last 35 years. In 1985, 64 percent of all women ages 16–64 were working for pay. More than 99 percent of teachers, 96 percent of nurses, 85 percent of librarians, 18 percent of lawyers, 21 percent of chemists, 15 percent of geologists, 11 percent of architects, and 8 percent of physicists are women.
- Only about 20 percent of the Americans receiving Ph.D.s in mathematics are women.
- In 1984, the starting salary for computer scientists, a common career choice among science majors, was $24,500; for chemical engineers, it was $27,000. The average salary offer to a student with a humanities background was under $18,000.
- More than one-third of families headed by females live below the poverty level.
- College-bound girls lag behind boys on the mathematics section of the Scholastic Aptitude Test by approximately 50 points.
- Forty percent of college-bound males enroll in three or more years of high school math; only 28 percent of college-bound females do.
- Women today on the average earn considerably less than their male counterparts who have the same education and experience.
- Of the 1,428 members in the National Academy of Science, only 53 are women.
- In the 1986 International Chemistry and Physics Olympiads, the American team members placed 23rd and 34th in the chemistry event while West Germany, East Germany, the U.S.S.R., and China garnered some of the highest awards. In the physics event, two gold medals went to Rumania and one to the U.S.S.R.; of the 10 silver and 14 bronze medals awarded, the American team received only three bronzes.

9. Find out about the following. If possible, view actual examples. Find some way of sharing your information.

- Holography
- Superconductors
- Fiber optics
- Large array radio telescopes
- Computer software
- Computer graphics
- Nuclear power generators
- Robotics

1. Who is a scientist? Describe the characteristics of a "typical" scientist. Younger girls may want to draw pictures of scientists and then describe their drawings. All the girls should have an opportunity to give their impressions of what scientists are like. Discuss the reasons why particular traits were selected. Were there strong similarities in the girls' descriptions? What would the group's composite scientist be like? Find examples of real people who are working in the sciences and compare impressions with reality.

2. There have been in the past and there are currently many renowned scientists and mathematicians who are women. Prepare a display, scrapbook, play, or biography about one or more of these women. The following list can help get you started.

- Emmy Noether
- Hypatia
- Trotula
- Anna Comnena
- Caroline Herschel
- Julia Robinson
- Sally Ride
- Barbara McClintock
- Sofya Kovalevskaya
- Margaret Knight
- Emily Roebling
- Marie Curie
- Evelyn Boyd Collins
- Grace Murray Hopper
- Rosalyn Yalow
- Rachel Carson
- Rosalind Franklin
- Marie Dolciani

3. Invite one or more women whose work is related to mathematics, science, or technology to a troop or group meeting. Be prepared to ask questions related not only to their present work but how they prepared for their careers, and what help or obstacles they found on the way.

4. Interview at least four women whose work is related to mathematics, science, or technology. Find out why each chose her job and what special actions she had to take to reach her career goals.

5. Develop a career file for jobs related to mathematics, science, and technology. Find some way to share this information with others. For example, you might use the file to help organize a career fair.

6. See mathematics, science, and technology in action. Plan an outing to a local business that uses or specializes in science, mathematics, or technology.

GSUSA Program Links

Note: The following program links are diverse because so many aspects of life relate to science and mathematics. While the World of Today and Tomorrow focuses specifically on science and math, activities from the other worlds of interest may also involve scientific and mathematical principles.

For All Girl Scouts

Exploring Wildlife Communities with Children (1981); Outdoor Education in Girl Scouting (1984). GSUSA Contemporary Issues: Be Your Best, Developing Health and Fitness (1992); Earth Matters, A Challenge for Environmental Action (1990).

For Daisy Girl Scouts

Daisy Girl Scouts Leaders' Guide
The Worlds of Interest: "The World of Today and Tomorrow" and "The World of the Arts" activities.

Exploring Wildlife Communities with Children

For Brownie Girl Scouts

Brownie Girl Scout Handbook (1993)
"How and Why" chapter. *Brownie Girl Scout Try-Its:* Animals, Building Art, Careers, Colors and Shapes, Creative Composing, Earth and Sky, Earth Is Our Home, Hobbies, Math Fun, Me and My Shadow, Movers, My Body, Numbers and Shapes, Outdoor Adventurer, Outdoor Fun, Outdoor Happenings, Plants, Science in Action, Science Wonders, Senses, Sound of Music.

National Science Partnership Kits (1993): Movers, Science Wonders, Space Explorers. (Available through NSP training for leaders. See description under *For Adults.*)

For Junior Girl Scouts

Junior Girl Scout Handbook (1994)
Chapter 4, "Skills to Use Every Day"; Chapter 5, "Everyone Is Different", Chapter 7, Exploring Interests, Skills and Talents." Badges: Careers, Discovering, Technology, Girls Are Great, Healthy Living, Science Discovery, Talk, Your Outdoor Surroundings, Science Is All Around You, My Natural Environment.

Girl Scout Badges and Signs (1990)
World of Well-Being: Across Generations, Exploring Healthy Eating, First Aid, Health and Fitness, Hobbies, Making Decisions, Sports, Sports Sampler. World of People: Creative Solutions, Geography Fun, Women's Stories, Women Today, World Neighbors. World of Today and Tomorrow: Dabbler, Aerospace, Business-Wise, Car Care, Computer Fun, Do-It-Yourself, Foods, Fibers, and Farming, Geology, Math Whiz, Money Sense, Ms. Fix-It, Plants and Animals, Puzzlers, Ready for Tomorrow, Science in Action, Science in the Worlds, Science Sleuth, Sky Search, Water Wonders, Weather Watch. World of the Arts: Architecture, Communication Arts, Drawing and Painting, Photography, Prints and Graphics, Video Production. World of the Out-of-Doors: Dabbler, Eco-Action, Ecology, Outdoor Cook, Outdoor Creativity, Outdoor Fun in the City, Walking for Fitness.

Junior Girl Scout Activity Book (1992): "Healthy Eating and Fitness"; "Discovering Science and Technology"; "Exploring the Natural World."

Natural Science Partnership Kits: Science Sleuth, Science in the Worlds, Weather Watch, Water Wonders. (Available through NSP training for leaders. See description under *For Adults* section.)

For Cadette and Senior Girl Scouts

Cadette and Senior Girl Scout Interest Projects (1987)
World of Well-Being: Dabbler, Collecting, Creative Cooking, Emergency Preparedness, Family Living, Fashion/Fitness/Makeup, Managing Stress, Pets, Skills for Living, Sports, Tune In to Well-Being. World of People: Dabbler, American Indian Lore, Community Time Capsule, Do You Get the Message?, Global Understanding, Heritage Hunt, Travel, Understanding Yourself and Others, Women's History. World of Today and Tomorrow: Dabbler, Audiovisual Production—Basic, Audiovisual Production—Advanced, Auto Maintenance, Career Exploration, Computers, Energy Awareness, Entrepreneurship, Geology, High-Tech Communication, Money Management, Plant Culture, Space Exploration. World of the Arts: Fashion Design and Clothing, Prints and Graphics, Visual Arts, Photography. World of the Out-of-Doors: Dabbler, Animal Observation, Backpacking, Camping, Eco-Action, Orienteering, Outdoor Survival, Paddle, Pole, and Roll, Skiing and Snowshoeing, Smooth Sailing, Water Sports, Wildlife.

Cadette and Senior Girl Scout Handbook (1995)
Chapter 3, "A Strength of One's Own: Developing Self-Esteem and a Healthy Lifestyle," Chapter 5, "Fun for Your Free Time," Chapter 6, "Skills for Life."

Senior Girl Scout Handbook (1995)
Chapter 4, "Careers of the Future," Chapter 5, "Skills for Living."

For Adults

Gender Equity Module, Ensuring Unbiased Behavior in an All-Girl Environment. GSUSA 1994. Training that can be delivered by council trainers.

National Science Partnership leader training modules, leader guides, and activity kits. NSP leader training consists of an introductory module for use in service units, along with seven training modules based upon three Brownie and four Junior Girl Scout science badges. Each kit has a leader's guide. Each kit provides materials for 15 girls for five to seven activity sessions. Kits and training were developed by The Franklin Institute Science Museum and GSUSA under a National Science Foundation Grant. Kits cost from $20 to $30 each. Councils are encouraged to work in partnership with science institutions to develop leader training and seek funding for kits.

"Reach for the Stars," (1993). National Science Partnership Video training to accompany NSP leader training on Space Explorer Kit for Brownie Girl Scouts.

"Weather Watch" (1994). National Science Partnership video to accompany NSP leader training on Weather Watch Kit for Junior Girl Scouts.

You and COMPUTERS

IT'S ELEMENTARY!

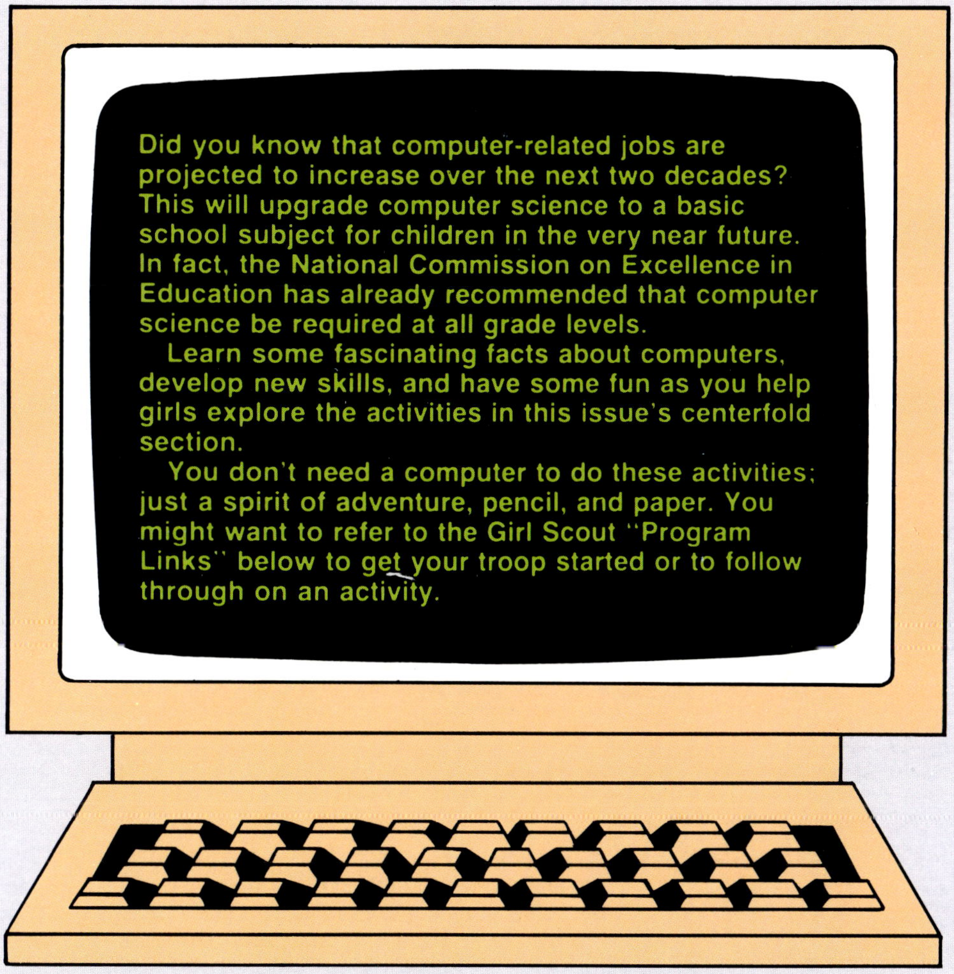

Why are computers called logic machines? Computers use logic in a step-by-step approach to arrive at conclusions. When given a set of true statements of facts or events, the computer processes the information and arrives at its logical conclusion. Consider the following statements:

Monday is the day before Tuesday.
Tuesday is always followed by Wednesday.
Today is Tuesday.
Therefore. . .

Using logical reasoning, it can be concluded that yesterday was Monday and tomorrow will be Wednesday.

Many everyday observations and events follow a logical sequence of actions and reactions. The ability to organize thoughts and ideas logically is an essential skill in writing computer programs. By observing and describing the order of events in your daily life, you can gain an understanding of the process involved in writing a computer program.

Think of two or more related true statements based on personal experiences and observations, and determine a logical conclusion. It might look like this:

Small pieces of dry wood will burn.
Tinder are small pieces of dry wood.
Therefore, tinder will burn.

Or this:

All Girl Scouts accept the Promise and Law.
Diana is a Girl Scout.
Therefore, Diana has accepted the Promise and Law.

Remember, the statements may relate to any experience you've had. Write down your ideas and share them with one another. Discuss why computers are called logic machines. Talk about the other uses for logical thinking.

Now that you have explored the concept of logic, you may be curious about how computers actually organize information. A computer uses a form of mathematical logic called Boolean logic. All the functions it performs are designed to require simple "yes" or "no" and "true" or "false" choices. The computer is programmed with the necessary information to determine its choices.

The game of 20 Questions is an example of Boolean logic.

One girl thinks of a subject that is either animal, vegetable, or mineral. The others try to guess its identity by asking questions that must be worded to require a "yes" or "no" answer. If a question cannot be answered with a simple "yes" or "no", the girl should respond, "It does not compute." By keeping a record of the questions and answers, you will have a visual record of how you arrived at the answer through Boolean logic.

COMPUTERESE

Computerese is a term used by some people in the computer field to describe the language that has developed as part of the new technology. This language includes technical and slang words, like the term 'computerese', which describe computers, how they work, what they can do, what you do with them, and so on. For example, a computer that is not functioning properly may produce incorrect information. This information may be referred to as "garbage" in computerese. The error in the computer program which may be keeping it from working properly is called a "bug."

Part of learning about computers is learning to speak their "language." Here are a few word games to help you get acquainted with computer terms (These words are listed below). You may decide to visit a library or computer store or invite a guest speaker to learn about these words.

WORD FIND

Fifteen computer words are hidden in the square below. See how many you can find. The words may be spelled from left to right, right to left, up or down, and on a diagonal. When you find a word, circle its letters; the first word has been circled for you. (Note: Some words share the same letters.)

E	E	R	R	O	R	M	E	S	S	A	G	E	X	E	F
R	B	S	K	D	J	G	M	P	H	C	I	S	T	X	L
A	I	A	C	C	U	M	U	L	A	T	O	R	P	J	O
W	N	I	P	B	D	E	K	I	U	W	T	C	U	Q	P
T	A	P	E	R	T	G	X	P	M	M	N	I	R	Y	P
F	R	D	B	U	D	V	N	E	B	E	R	S	R	A	Y
O	Y	V	C	F	S	I	J	L	S	M	V	A	E	G	D
S	R	E	T	U	P	M	O	C	W	O	F	B	T	M	I
E	X	C	H	A	R	A	C	T	E	R	Y	R	N	O	S
E	L	B	A	I	R	A	V	J	O	Y	S	T	I	C	K

ACCUMULATOR
BASIC
BINARY
CHARACTER
COMPUTER
DEBUG
ERROR MESSAGE
EXECUTE
FLOPPY DISK
INPUT
INTERRUPT
JOYSTICK
MEMORY
SOFTWARE
VARIABLE

COMPUTER TERMS

Creating word games can be hours of fun! You can challenge your friends by using your scrambled word sets, coded words, or Word Find gameboards. Here are some computer terms from which to choose, and directions for making a Word Find gameboard.

ACOUSTIC COUPLER	CHARACTER	DEBUG	HARDWARE
ACCUMULATOR	CHIP	DISK	INPUT
ALPHANUMERIC	CODE	END OF FILE (EOF)	INTERRUPT
BASIC	COMPUTER	ERROR MESSAGE	JOYSTICK
BINARY	COMPILER	ESCAPE KEY	KEYBOARD
BIT	C.R.T. (Cathode Ray Tube)	EXECUTE	LIBRARY
BUG		FIELD	LOOP
BYTE	CURSOR	FILE	MEMORY
C.P.U. (Central Processing Unit)	DAISY WHEEL	FLOPPY DISK	MENU
	DATA	FORMAT	MICROCOMPUTER

D·E·C·O·D·E· A ·W·O·R·D

A computer with a "bug" in its program has produced this "garbage"—a list of nonsense words. The programmer discovered that the computer has incorrectly coded the letters of the alphabet. For instance, each time it was meant to print the letter A, it printed the letter V in its place. Can you help the programmer decode this computer?

(Hint: These words are included in the list of computer terms on page 16. Start by writing the letter A everywhere you see the letter V.)

MVIV = _ _ _ _

NVEMOVEU = _ _ _ _ _ _ _ _ _ _

DUDFEL = _ _ _ _ _ _ _

JFEDVI = _ _ _ _ _ _ _

TFFZ = _ _ _ _

ZVYYOFEM = _ _ _ _ _ _ _ _ _ _

SCRAMBLED WORDS

Unscramble the letters to find four basic computer terms. Arrange the letters in correct order and write one letter in each box.

O D E C

U N E M

D R C O R E

P O U T T U

Now that you're finished, try unscrambling the circled letters to answer this question:

QUESTION: What plays games, counts, remembers facts, and rarely makes a mistake?

ANSWER:

A

GIRL SCOUT *Mystery* WORD GAME

Learn computer terms while playing the mystery word game. Choose a girl to act as the "word processor" and ask her to pick a mystery word. Take turns trying to guess a letter in the word. When a letter guessed in the mystery word is correct, the player may try to guess the word. For every incorrect guess, the word processor writes a letter in the words "Girl Scout." The game is over when a player correctly identifies the word or the word processor completely spells Girl Scout.

(Note: Keep a list of the incorrect letters named to avoid repetition.)

MODEM
OUTPUT
PASSWORD
PLOTTER
PRINTER
PROGRAM
RECORD
SOFTWARE
VARIABLE
WORD PROCESSOR

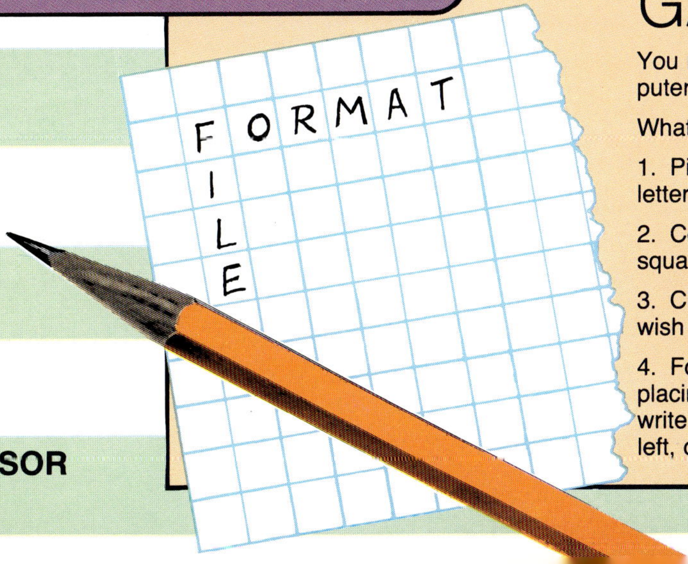

WORD FIND GAMEBOARD

You need: graph paper, pencil, computer terms

What to do:

1. Pick a starting box, and write the letter X inside.
2. Count 15 squares across and 15 squares down from the starting box.
3. Choose the computer terms you wish to include on the gameboard.
4. Form words on the board by placing a letter in each box. You can write them from left to right, right to left, on a diagonal, and up or down.

Girls Plus Math Equal Fun

World of Well-Being

The Inside Story

Many signs of health and well-being are measured in numbers. Your body temperature, pulse (heart rate), and respiration (breathing rate) are three vital signs you can learn to measure and understand. Your temperature will measure no more than a few degrees above or below 98.6°F, unless you are not feeling well. Your heart rate and breathing depends on what you are doing. Find out how to measure your body temperature, heart rate, and respiration; learn what makes them change.

You will need a thermometer, a watch with a second hand, and a pencil and paper to record the measurements. Before starting the activity, read these directions and practice them a few times. Then record your vital numbers.

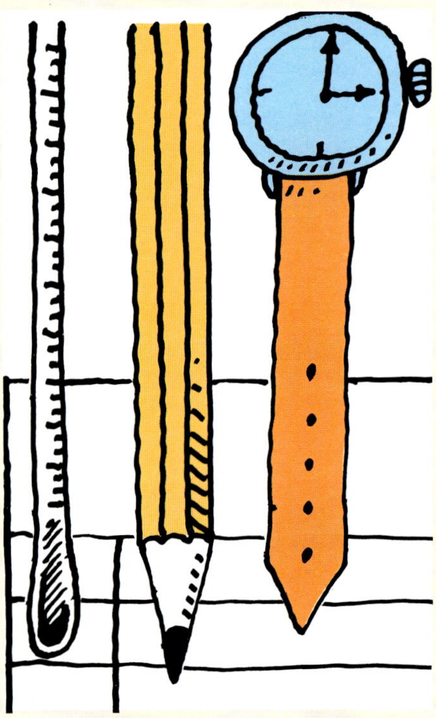

Taking your temperature Place a clean thermometer that reads less than 96° under your tongue and leave it there for at least three minutes. Remove the thermometer and find the number where the mercury stopped.

Taking your pulse Place two fingers on the side of your neck and move them about slowly until you feel your pulse—a thumping movement. Each thump is a heartbeat. Look at the second hand on your watch and count the number of thumps you feel in 30 seconds. Double this number to get your heart rate.

Taking your breathing rate Ask someone to count the number of times you breathe in in 30 seconds. Double this number to get your breathing rate.

Lie down with your eyes closed for five minutes. Then measure your temperature, pulse, and respiration rate, and record the figures. Do two simple activities—walking for five minutes, jumping 15 times—and measure your three vital signs after each. Look at the numbers you recorded and discuss what made some of them change.

*Find out how to measure other vital signs, such as your blood pressure and lung capacity, and learn about the activities that make the numbers change.

Make a Life Line

You learned to do different things at different ages. When did you learn to crawl, to walk, to talk? Make a record of events as they happened in your life.

You will need index cards, paper, ruler, yarn or string, and crayons. Write an important event in your life on each card and how old you were when it happened, such as ''I started to crawl,'' ''I got my first tooth,'' ''I spoke my first words.'' You will probably need to ask an older family member for help. Draw a picture on each card and use string or yarn to connect them in the right order. Then have fun comparing your life line with others.

*Link your past, present, and future by showing the events in your life on a time line. Make every month of your life equal one centimeter or one inch. The beginning of your life line might look like the drawing below.

Include events that you think might happen as you get older. Compare your time line with others.

Counting Calories

Calories are a measure of heat energy. They show how much energy you need to use up to equal the amount of food you eat. If you ''fuel up'' and eat more calories than you ''burn up,'' your body stores the extra calories and gains weight. If you use up more energy than the fuel you take in, you lose weight.

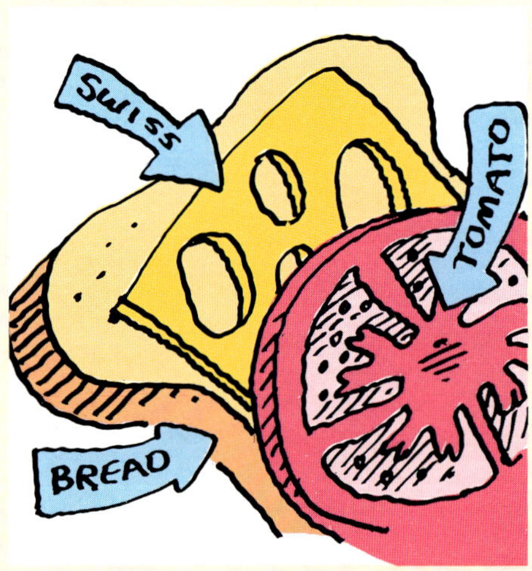

Find out the calorie count of the food you eat. Make a list of high, moderate, and low calorie foods.

*Plan a meal or snack and list the calorie count of each item on the menu.

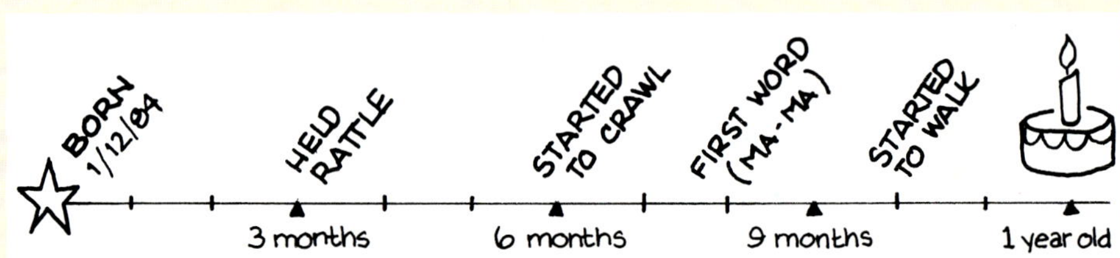

World of People

Measure Up

People around the world developed different systems for measuring. For example, centuries ago in England a foot was based on the length of a man's foot. Since not everyone had the same size foot, this led to confusion. Now the measure called one foot means the same to everyone: 12 inches.

In most countries today, people use the metric system, but in the United States, most people still use what is called the English system.

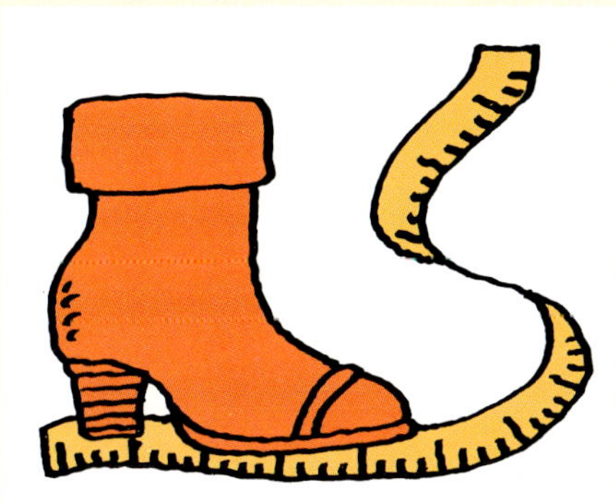

Practice measuring objects with the tools of each system—a ruler, a meter stick, a measuring cup, a liter container. For example, measure the length of a book in centimeters and then in inches. The book doesn't change—but the numbers do.

*Make a chart comparing the metric system and the English system we use.

1 teaspoon = 5 milliliters
1 quart = .956 liters
1 inch = 2½ centimeters

What other comparisons can you make?

Money Matters

Money or currency is used around the world in exchange for goods and services. In our country the dollar is the basic unit of currency. It is based on the number

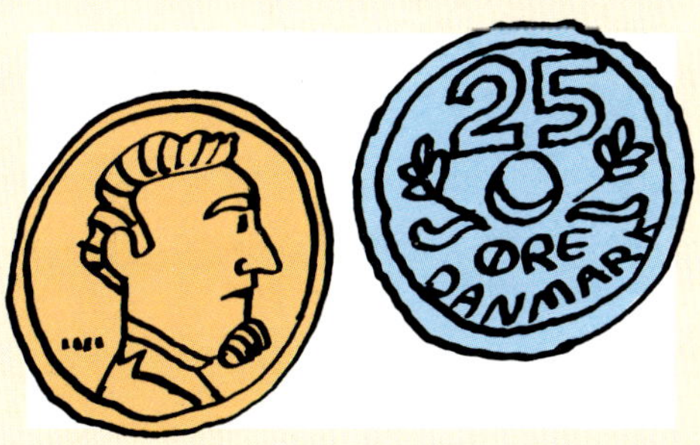

10 and its symbol is the dollar sign. One dollar is written $1.00.

Other countries use different basic units and symbols for their currencies. Visit a library or coin-exchange store to learn about them. For example, in Mexico the basic unit is called a peso and the symbol used is $; in Japan the basic unit is the yen and the symbol is Y. Look at samples of money from other countries and compare them to U.S. money.

*Use this chart to see about how much one U.S. dollar is worth in other currencies. For example, $1.00 is worth 51 francs in Belgium. How much is it worth in the other countries listed? Figure out how much your troop treasury would be worth in each country.

Currency Exchange Rates
(September 1983)

Country	*Unit Symbol*	*Currency Equivalents (in one U.S. dollar)*
United States	Dollar $	1.00
Belgium	Franc Fr	51.00
China	Renminbi	2.00
Greece	Drachma Dr	84.00
India	Rupee Re	10.00
Italy	Lire L	1460.00
Japan	Yen Y	233.00
Mexico	Peso $	140.00
Portugal	Escudo $ (or Esc)	110.00

Setting It Up

Objects with something in common make up a set. Some of them may also belong to another, smaller set called a subset. For example, everyone belongs to the human race, but they are also members of different subsets—such as people with blue eyes, people with brown eyes, and so on.

Girl Scout recognitions can be grouped into sets. One set of Girl Scout badges has five subsets—badges in the World of Well-Being, the World of People, the World of Today and Tomorrow, the World of the Arts, and the World of the Out-of-Doors.

Make up five of your own sets. You could collect pictures or make drawings to illustrate them. What do the members of each set have in common?

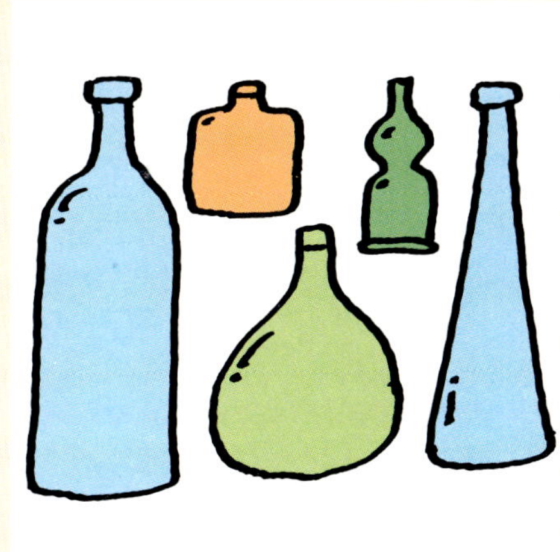

*Make up five sets with at least two subsets each. An example would be a set of animals with four legs. Two subsets could be animals with scaly skin and animals with fur.

World of Today and Tomorrow

Marking Time

Keeping track of time is important to people. Sand clocks (hourglasses) and sundials were two of the earliest clocks invented. Each depended on elements of nature for keeping track of time. Find out how well they worked by following these directions for marking time.

Hourglass (Sand clock)

You will need two dry, glass jars of the same size, heavy paper, pencil, masking tape, scissors, a nail or pin, sand or salt, and a watch.

Trace the mouth of one jar on the heavy paper. Cut out the circle and punch a hole in its center using the nail or pin. Pour sand or salt into one jar, filling it almost to the top. Place the paper circle over the filled jar. Next, put the empty jar on top of the filled jar and cardboard circle. (Make sure the mouth of the jar is touching the cardboard.) Carefully tape the jars together to make a seal. You now have a clock. Turn the clock over and record the time it takes to empty the top jar. You can adjust your clock by making the hole in the cardboard larger or smaller and by changing the amount of sand or salt used.

*Sundial (Shadow clock)

You will need a pencil (about 4 inches long) with an eraser, heavy paper or cardboard (8½″ × 11″), a thumbtack, a telephone book, tape, a compass, a pencil to write with, and a sunny day.

Mark the middle of the paper or

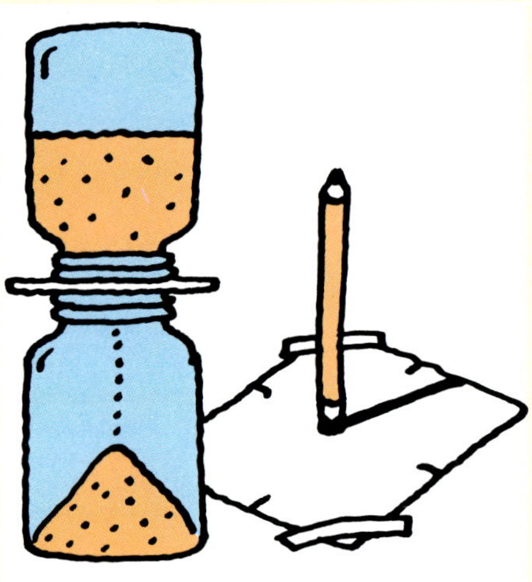

cardboard along one of its long sides. Push the thumbtack through this mark with the point sticking up. Tape the corners of the paper in place. Push the pencil eraser down over the point, making sure the pencil is as straight as you can get it. You now have the beginnings of a sundial.

Pick an open, level spot outside to set your sundial on a sunny day. Try to start early in the morning. Find north with your compass and position the sundial so that the pencil is facing north. The shadow of the pencil should fall on the paper. Check your sundial every hour and trace the shadow made by the pencil on the paper. Record the hour at the tip of each shadow tracing. At the end of the day, connect the tips with a line. What shape does the line make?

Testing 1-2-3

Probability is a number prediction of whether something might happen. It is more accurate than a guess, but may not always be true. Try it for yourself:

■ If you flipped a penny 20 times, how often will it land on its head?

■ Flip a penny 10 times and tally how many times it lands on heads and on tails. Do this 10 more times. Compare the results after 20 flips. Is a pattern emerging?

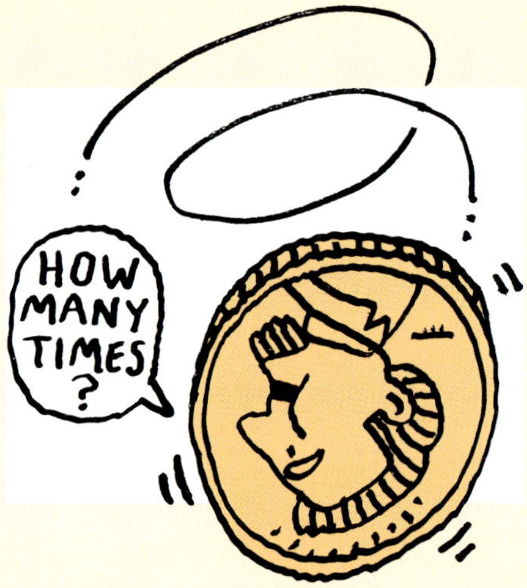

■ Try flipping the penny a total of 100 times. Make sure you tally each flip on a chart. Can you now predict how many times you will get heads if you flip a quarter 30 times?

*ABCs

What letter of the alphabet is used most often?

Pick five sentences from a book and count how many times each letter is used. Based on your findings, try to predict the letter that will show up most often in any particular sentence. Test your prediction.

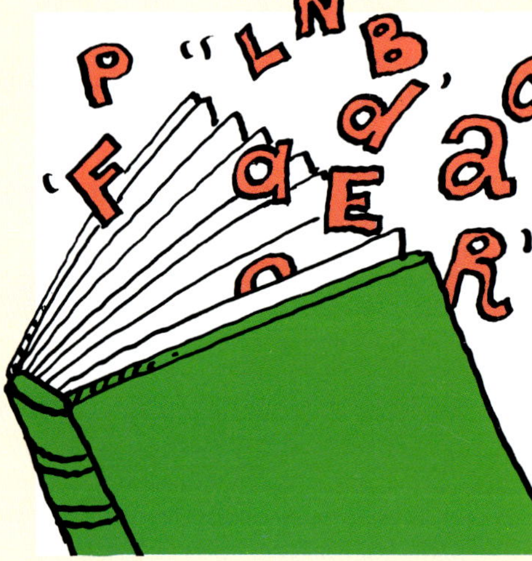

■ If there were two red balls and one blue ball in a paper bag, what is the chance of picking two red balls?

*The Ballgame

You need two red balls and one blue ball or marbles and a paper bag. Put the balls in the bag and shake. Close your eyes and pick out two balls. Are they the same color or different? What happens in 25 tries? Keep a chart to learn the probabilities.

Mobius Twists

Every piece of paper has two flat surfaces. A mobius twist has only one continuous flat surface. To make a mobius twist, cut a strip of paper one inch wide and at least 10 inches long and follow the directions in the drawings.

You can show the two separate sides of the loop by placing a pen in the inside center of the simple loop and drawing a line on the surface. Only the inside will have a line. Now try this with the mobius twist. You should end up with one continuous line on all surfaces.

Cut the two paper loops in half lengthwise. When you cut the simple loop, you get two thinner loops. What happens when you cut the mobius twist?

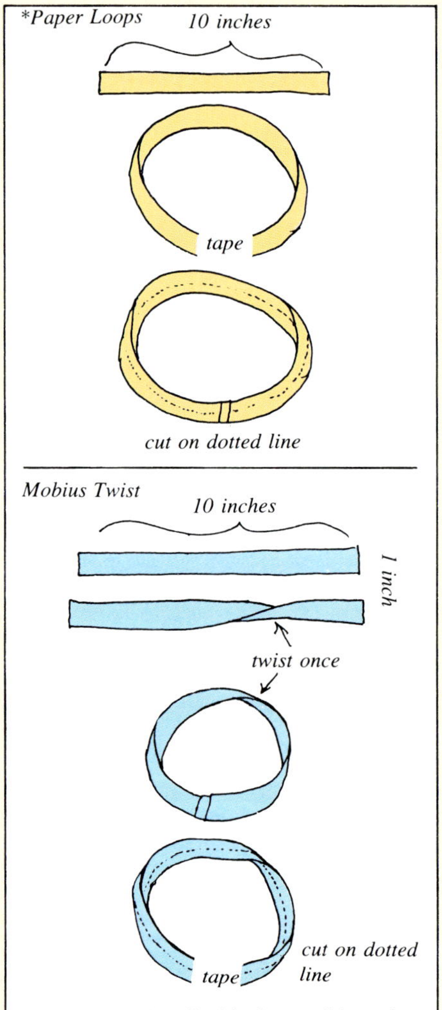

Start the cut described in the asterisk section here.
After one circular cut, continue to cut the last two thirds in half.

*Ready for more mobius magic? Start with a fresh mobius twist. Cut in ⅓ of the way from the edge and continue cutting. What do you get?

World of the Arts

Colors

You can create a whole range of colors from the three primary colors of red, blue, and yellow—and even more by adding black or white. Learn about proportions as you mix different paints to get different colors.

You will need five jars of tempera paint (red, yellow, blue, black, and white), five eye droppers, an aluminum pie plate or squares of wax paper, a paintbrush, and a container of water.

Begin by choosing two colors and add one drop of each to the pie plate or paper. (Use different eye droppers for each color.)

Mix the colors with the paint brush. What color do you have? Make a chart to record what happened after each drop.

Do this with other pairs of colors. Make sure the paintbrush and mixing surface are clean before starting. Paint a picture with the colors you made.

*Paint a color wheel, showing complementary colors.

Sounds

Sound waves are produced by vibrations. Different sounds can be made by changing the object that is vibrating. For example, the sound made by a vibrating rubber band will change as it is stretched longer and narrower. Try the following activity to make different sounds.

You will need eight identical glass containers (bottles, jars, or glasses), a spoon, and water. Place the glasses about two inches apart in a straight line on a table. Tap each lightly with the spoon. The sounds made by the air vibrating in the glasses should be similar.

Now pour the same amount of water into two glasses. Tap each one again. What happened?

Add water to all eight glasses, putting a little more in each one. Tap each glass, starting with the one that has the least amount of water. What do you hear?

*Play a simple tune by tapping the glasses. Remember how you can change the sounds.

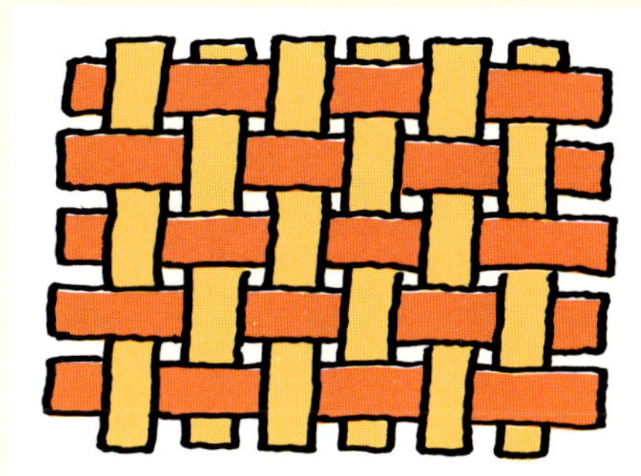

Patterns

A pattern is formed when something is repeated in a regular sequence. The number pattern 123123123 is easy to complete because it follows a sequence. Numerical patterns are used to plan other kinds of patterns. For example, in the textile industry, weaving looms are programmed using numbers to represent colors. You can create your own program to make color patterns.

You will need strips of paper in two or more colors, each about 11 inches long and one inch wide; cardboard or heavy paper about 10 inches wide; and tape or glue.

Place strips of one color side-by-side on the cardboard to cover it completely. Fold the cardboard and tape them to the back. Thread the second color through the strips, working over and under on one line, then under and over on the next.

When you have finished, describe what you see by moving across one row of strips and calling out the colors. What is your color pattern? What is the last color in the row? What color would come next?

*Try weaving a pattern using three or more colors or three different threading techniques.

Collect scraps of fabric to make a quilt wall hanging. What pattern will you use in your design?

*World of the Out-of-Doors

Symmetry

When two halves of an object are identical, the object has bilateral symmetry. Many animals and plants are symmetrical.

Use an imaginary line to cut an object in half. Compare each side. Are they the same? If so, the object has bilateral symmetry; if not, it is asymmetrical. Take your imaginary line with you on a hunt for symmetry in nature.

*Although your face has bilateral symmetry, the right and left halves are not exactly identical. You can see this by looking in the mirror and covering half your face. Do you see any slight

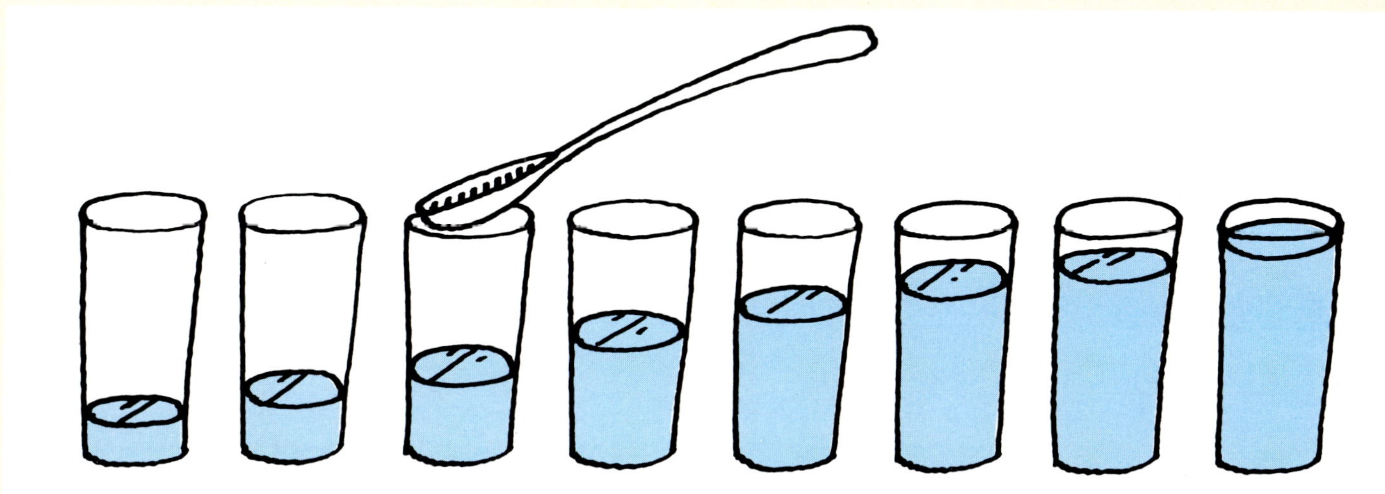

differences in the two halves?

*Some objects look the same from all sides. They have rotational symmetry. Look for natural and man-made objects in your neighborhood with rotational symmetry.

Shaping Up

Circles, triangles, squares, and rectangles are geometric shapes. Many things in nature have geometric shapes. The iris (colored part) of your eye is a circle,

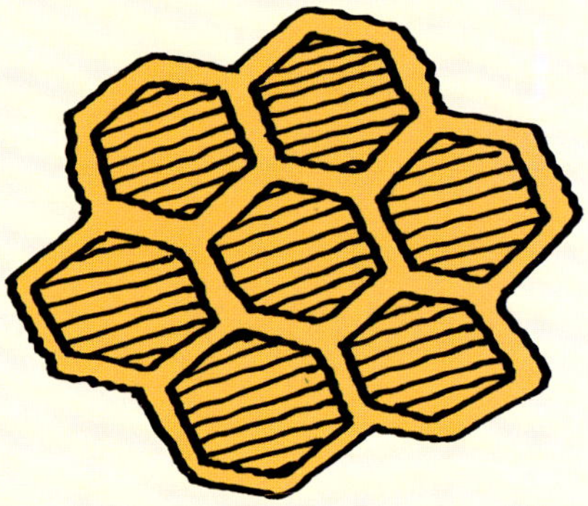

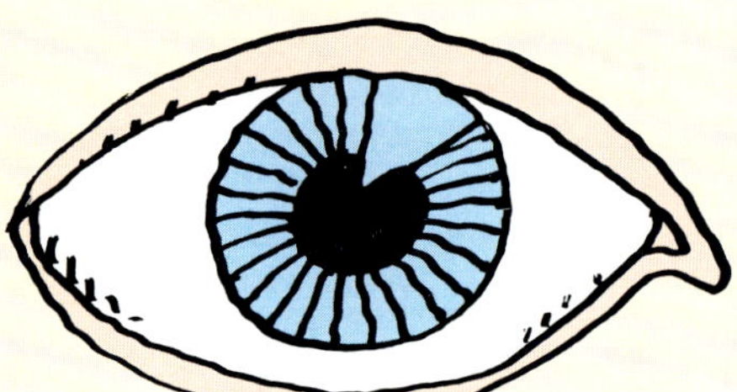

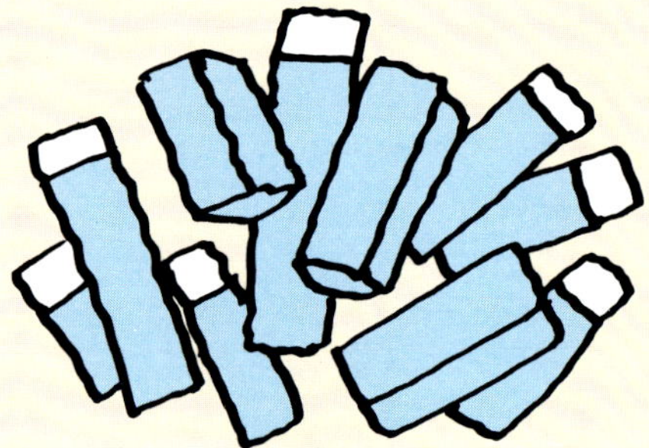

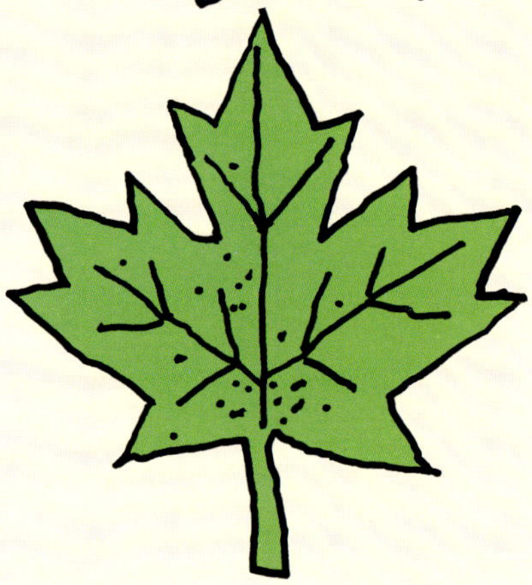

salt crystals form in squares, and the spaces in a beehive are hexagons (6 sides).

Find out how things around your town shape up. Make a chart of shapes to look for before starting out. You may also want to carry a magnifying glass to examine small objects—such as crystals in rocks and stones. Record the objects you find on your chart, and draw pictures of them. Leave space on the chart to add extra shapes you may discover along the way.

Natural Numbers

Numbers help people identify objects in nature. All insects have six legs. Poison ivy has three leaves on each stem, and a maple leaf has five main points.

Discover more about numbers in nature. Find out what other plants and animals can be identified because of numbers.

*Many organisms have striking mathematical characteristics. Look for the opposite spirals in a pine cone and a pineapple. What other interesting patterns can you discover in nature?

—Sharon Woods Hussey
and Damariz Z. Winborne

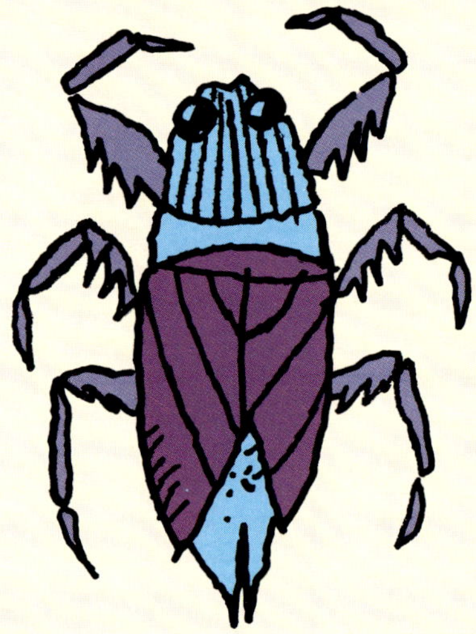

Sharon Woods Hussey is director of GSUSA's Program Department; Damariz Z. Winborne is a program specialist in the department.

Word Game Solutions

WORD FIND

E	E	R	R	O	R	M	E	S	S	A	G	E	X	E	F
R	B	S	K	D	J	G	M	P	H	C	I	S	T	X	L
A	I	A	C	C	U	M	U	L	A	T	O	R	P	J	O
W	N	I	P	B	D	E	K	I	U	W	T	C	U	Q	P
T	A	P	E	R	T	G	X	P	M	M	N	I	R	Y	P
F	R	D	B	U	D	V	N	E	B	E	R	S	R	A	Y
O	Y	V	C	F	S	I	J	L	S	M	V	A	E	G	D
S	R	E	T	U	P	M	O	C	W	O	F	B	T	M	I
E	X	C	H	A	R	A	C	T	E	R	Y	R	N	O	S
E	L	B	A	I	R	A	V	J	O	Y	S	T	I	C	K

SCRAMBLED WORD
O D E C is CODE
U N E M is MENU
D R C O R E is RECORD
P O U T T U is OUTPUT
C O M U E R P T is COMPUTER

DECODE A WORD

Letter Key: A = V, D = M, E = U, F = J, H = N, L = T, M = D, O = F, P = Z, R = E, S = Y, T = I, W = O, Y = L

Word List: M V I V is DATA
N V E M O V E U is HARDWARE
D U D F E L is MEMORY
J F E D V I is FORMAT
T F F Z is LOOP
Z V Y Y O F E M is PASSWORD

Resources

Local Sources

On the following pages is a comprehensive list of mathematics, science, and technology resources that are available on a national basis. However, before you turn to such sources, you may want to thoroughly explore what is available in your own backyard. The following checklist can assist you in identifying all the local possibilities that you will probably want to try first.

Schools, educational community:
- School counselors
- Mathematics and science teachers, or department chairs
- Curriculum coordinators
- Local community college or university
- Libraries
- Girl Scout council office. (Your local Girl Scout council has a special videotape that highlights how Girl Scout leaders can use "Square One," produced by Children's Television Workshop, to stimulate girls' interest in math.)

Business and industry, community organizations:
- Chamber of Commerce
- Local businesses
- Civic clubs and organizations
- Science editor of a local newspaper
- Museums, nature centers, zoos

Federal agencies with local offices in the community:
- Bureau of Land Management
- U.S. Forest Service
- Soil Conservation Service
- U.S. Army Corps of Engineers
- Military bases
- National Park Service
- U.S. Fish and Wildlife Service
- U.S. Weather Bureau

National Organizations Related to Mathematics, Science, and Technology

Alpha Epsilon Delta
University of Virginia
Garrett Hall
Charlottesville, Va. 22904

American Academy of Arts and Sciences
136 Irving Street
Cambridge, Mass. 02138

American Academy of Forensic Sciences
218 E. Cache La Poudre
P.O. Box 669
Colorado Springs, Colo. 80901-0669

American Academy of Optometry
5530 Wisconsin Avenue, N.W., Suite 1149
Washington, D.C. 20815

American Anthropological Association
1703 New Hampshire Avenue, N.W.
Washington, D.C. 20009

American Association for the Advancement of Science
1333 H Street, N.W.
Washington, D.C. 20005

American Association for Dental Research
1111 14th Street, N.W., #1000
Washington, D.C. 20005

American Association of Blacks in Energy
801 Pennsylvania Avenue, S.E., Suite 250
Washington, D.C. 20003

American Association of Colleges of Pharmacy
1426 Prince Street
Alexandria, Va. 22314

American Association of Dental Schools
1625 Massachusetts Avenue, N.W.
Washington, D.C. 20036

American Association of Immunologists
Committee on Women's Affairs
9650 Rockville Pike
Bethesda, Md. 20014

American Association of Petroleum Geologists
P.O. Box 979
Tulsa, Okla. 74101

American Association of Physics Teachers
5112 Berwyn Road
College Park, Md. 20740

American Association of University Professors
1012 14th Street, N.W., #500
Washington, D.C. 20005

American Association of University Women
1111 Sixteenth Street, N.W.
Washington, D.C. 20036

American Association of Women Dentists (AAWD)
111 E. Wacker Drive, Suite 600
Chicago, Ill. 60601

American Astronomical Society
c/o Dr. Peter B. Boyce
2000 Florida Avenue, N.W., #300
Washington, D.C. 20009

American Chemical Society
Women Chemists Committee
1155 16th Street, N.W.
Washington, D.C. 20036

American Dairy Science Association
c/o Carl D. Johnson
309 W. Clark Street
Champaign, Ill. 61820

American Dental Association
211 East Chicago Avenue
Chicago, Ill. 60611

American Dietetic Association
Division of Education and Research
216 W. Jackson Boulevard, Suite 800
Chicago, Ill. 60606

American Geographical Society
156 Fifth Avenue, #600
New York, N.Y. 10010

American Geological Institute
4220 King Street
Alexandria, Va. 22302

American Industrial Hygiene Association
P.O. Box 8390
345 White Pond Drive
Akron, Ohio 44320

American Institute of Aeronautics and Astronautics
Educational Programs
370 L'Enfant Promenade, S.W.
Washington, D.C. 20024

The American Institute of Architects
1735 New York Avenue, N.W.
Washington, D.C. 20011

American Institute of Biological Sciences
730 11th Street, N.W.
Washington, D.C. 20001-4584

American Institute of Chemical Engineers
345 East 47th Street
New York, N.Y. 10017

American Institute of Chemists
7315 Wisconsin Avenue, N.W.
Bethesda, Md. 20814

American Institute of Industrial Engineers (AIIE)
25 Technology Park/Atlanta
Norcross, Ga. 30092

American Institute of Physics
335 East 45th Street
New York, N.Y. 10017

American Institute of Professional Geologists
7828 Vance Drive, #103
Arvada, Colo. 80003

American Library Association
50 East Huron Street
Chicago, Ill. 60611

American Mathematical Society
P.O. Box 6248
Providence, R.I. 02940

Council on Medical Education of the American Medical Association
535 North Dearborn Street
Chicago, Ill. 60610

American Medical Women's Association
801 North Fairfax Street, Suite 400
Alexandria, Va. 22314

American Medical Writers Association
9650 Rockville Pike
Bethesda, Md. 20814

American Meteorological Society
45 Beacon Street
Boston, Mass. 02108

American Nature Study Society
c/o John A. Gustafson
5881 Cold Brook Rd.
Homer, N.Y. 13077

American Pharmaceutical Association
2215 Constitution Avenue, N.W.
Washington, D.C. 20037

American Physical Society
335 East 45th Street
New York, N.Y. 10017

American Physical Therapy Association
1111 North Fairfax Street
Alexandria, Va. 22314

American Physiological Society
9650 Rockville Pike
Bethesda, Md. 20814

American Psychological Association
1200 17th Street, N.W.
Washington, D.C. 20036

American Public Health Association
1015 15th Street, N.W.
Washington, D.C. 20005

American Society of Civil Engineers
345 East 47th Street
New York, N.Y. 10017

American Society of Ichthyologists and Herpetologists
Department of Zoology
Southern Illinois University
Carbondale, Ill. 62901-6501

American Society of Limnology and Oceanography
Virginia Institute of Marine Science
The College of William and Mary
Gloucester Point, Va. 23062

American Society of Mechanical Engineers
Education Services
345 East 47th Street
New York, N.Y. 10017

American Society of Zoologists
104 Sirius Circle
Thousand Oaks, Calif. 91360

American Statistical Association
1429 Duke Street
Alexandria, Va. 22314

Animal Behavior Society
Department of Psychology, CB 345
University of Colorado
Boulder, Colo. 80309

Archaeological Institute of America
675 Commonwealth Avenue
Boston, Mass. 02215

Association for Women in Mathematics
Wellesley College
106 Central Street
Wellesley, Mass. 02181

Association for Women in Psychology (AWP)
370 Lancaster Avenue
Haverford College
Haverford, Pa. 19041-1392

Association for Women in Science
2401 Virginia Avenue, N.W., Suite 303
Washington, D.C. 20037

Association for Women Veterinarians
c/o Chris Stone Payne, DVM
32205 Allison Drive
Union City, Calif. 94587

Association of Science and Technology Centers
1413 K Street, N.W., 10th Floor
Washington, D.C. 20005

Association of Women Geoscientists (AWG)
10200 W. 44th Avenue, Suite 304
Wheat Ridge, Colo. 80033

Association of Women in Computing, Inc.
P.O. Box 21100
St. Paul, Minn. 55123

Botanical Society of America
Ecology and Evolutionary Biology
75 N. Eagleville Road
U-43 University of Connecticut
Storrs, Conn. 06269-0043

Ecological Society of America
Center for Environmental Studies
Arizona State University
Tempe, Ariz. 85287

Entomological Society of America
9301 Annapolis Road
Lanham, Md. 20706-3115

Foundation for Science and the Handicapped
236 Grand Street
Morgantown, W.Va. 26505-7509

Geological Society of America
P.O. Box 9140
Boulder, Colo. 80301

History of Science Society
35 Dean Street
Worcester, Mass. 01609

Institute of Environmental Sciences
940 E. North-West Highway
Mt. Prospect, Ill. 60056

Institute of Food Technologists
221 N. LaSalle Street
Chicago, Ill. 60601

Junior Engineering Technical Society
1420 King Street, #405
Alexandria, Va. 22314

Mathematical Association of America
1529 18th Street, N.W.
Washington, D.C. 20036

Math/Science Network
2727 College Avenue
Berkeley, Calif. 94705

Medical Library Association
6 North Michigan Avenue, Suite 300
Chicago, Ill. 60602

National Association for Research in Science Teaching
c/o Glenn Markle
401 Teachers' College
University of Cincinnati
Cincinnati, Ohio 45221

National Association of Biology Teachers
11250 Roger Bacon Drive, #19
Reston, Va. 22090

National Association of Geology Teachers
c/o Dr. Robert Christman
Department of Geology
W. Washington University
Bellingham, Wash. 98225

National Association of Science Writers
P.O. Box 294
Greenlawn, N.Y. 11740

National Association for Geographic Education
16 A Leonard Hall
Indiana University of Pennsylvania
Indiana, Pa. 15705

National Council of Teachers of Mathematics
1906 Association Drive
Reston, Va. 22091

National Institute of Science
c/o Dr. Arthur C. Washington
P.O. Box 2784
Prairie View, Tex. 77446

National Network of Minority Women in Science
American Association for the Advancement of Science
1333 H. Street, N.W.
Washington, D.C. 20005

National Organization for the Professional Advancement of Black Chemists and Chemical Engineers
c/o Department of Chemistry
P.O. Box 5
Howard University
Washington, D.C. 20059

National Science Teachers Association
1742 Connecticut Avenue, N.W.
Washington, D.C. 20009

National Wildlife Federation
1400 16th Street, N.W.
Washington, D.C. 20036

Paleontological Society
c/o Donald Wolberg
New Mexico Bureau of Mines and Mineral Resources
Socorro, N.Mex. 87801

School Science and Mathematics Association
Bowling Green State University
126 Life Sciences
Bowling Green, Ohio 43403

Sigma Delta Epsilon
(Graduate Women in Science)
P.O. Box 4748
Ithaca, N.Y. 14852

Society for Environmental Geochemistry and Health
c/o Willard R. Chappell
Center for Environmental Sciences
Campus Box 136
University of Colorado
Denver, Colo. 80204

Society of American Foresters
5400 Grosvenor Lane
Bethesda, Md. 20814

Society of Women Engineers
United Engineering Center, Room 305
345 East 47th Street
New York, N.Y. 10017

Wildlife Management Institute
1101 14th Street, N.W., #725
Washington, D.C. 20005

Women and Mathematics Education (WME)
c/o Charlene Morrow
302 Shattuck Hall
Mount Holyoke College
S. Hadley, Mass. 01075

Women in Cell Biology
c/o Dr. Mina Bissell
Lawrence Berkeley Laboratory
Building 83/101
1 Cyclotron Road
Berkeley, Calif. 94720

Women in Mining
909 17th Street, Suite 418
Denver, Colo. 80202

New Entries

An Income of Her Own
406 Lion Street
Ojai, Calif. 93023

Securities Industry Foundation for Economic Education
Securities Industry Association
120 Broadway
New York, N.Y. 10271

Museums and Other Science Centers

Many museums throughout the country are dedicated to developing the public's knowledge and appreciation of science and technology. Below are some of them, listed by state. Those institutions starred (*) are National Science Partners.

Alabama

Alabama Space and Rocket Center
Tranquility Base
Huntsville, Ala. 35087

Anniston Museum of Natural History
4301 McClellan Boulevard
P.O. Box 1587
Anniston, Ala. 36202

The Discovery Place
1320 22nd Street South
Birmingham, Ala. 35205

The Exploreum
1906 Springhill Avenue
Mobile, Ala. 33607

Red Mountain Museum
1421 22nd Street South
Birmingham, Ala. 35205

Arizona

Arizona Museum of Science and Technology*
80 North 2nd Street
Phoenix, Ariz. 85004

The Human Adventure Center*
P.O. Box 31808
Tucson, Ariz. 85751

Museum of Northern Arizona*
Route 4, Box 720
Flagstaff, Ariz. 86001

Arkansas

Arkansas Museum of Science and History*
Mac Arthur Park
Little Rock, Ark. 72202

California

California Museum of Science and Industry*
700 State Drive
Exposition Park
Los Angeles, Calif. 90037

The Exploratorium
3601 Lyon Street
San Francisco, Calif. 94123

Lawrence Hall of Science
University of California
Berkeley, Calif. 94720

The Oakland Museum
1000 Oak Street
Oakland, Calif. 94607

Palo Alto Junior Museum
1451 Middlefield Road
Palo Alto, Calif. 94301

Reuben H. Fleet Space Theater and Science Center
1875 El Prado, Balboa Park
P.O. Box 33303
San Diego, Calif. 92103

San Francisco Bay Model Visitor Center
2100 Bridgeway Boulevard
Sausalito, Calif. 94965

Santa Barbara Museum of Natural History
2559 Puesta del Sol
Santa Barbara, Calif. 93105

Santa Barbara Science Discovery Center
813 State Street
Santa Barbara, Calif. 93101

Colorado

Colorado Science Center
P.O. Box 328
Denver, Colo. 80201

Hall of Life
Health Education Center
700 Broadway, Suite 114
Denver, Colo. 80273

Connecticut

Museum of Art, Science, and Industry, Inc.
4450 Park Avenue
Bridgeport, Conn. 06604

Science Museum of Connecticut*
950 Trout Brook Drive
West Hartford, Conn. 06119

Thames Science Center
Gallows Lane
New London, Conn. 06320

District of Columbia

Explorers Hall
National Geographic Society
17th and M Streets, N.W.
Washington, D.C. 20036

National Academy of Sciences
2101 Constitution Avenue, N.W.
Washington, D.C. 20418

National Air and Space Museum
James C. Tyler, Acting Director
Smithsonian Institution
6th and Independence Avenue, S.W.
Washington, D.C. 20560

National Museum of American History
Smithsonian Institution
12th Street and Constitution Avenue, N.W.
Washington, D.C. 20560

Florida

Discovery Center
231 S.W. 2nd Avenue
Ft. Lauderdale, Fla. 33301

The Habitat Museum
1450 Merrihue Drive
Naples, Fla. 33942

Jacksonville Museum of Arts and Sciences
1025 Gulf Life Drive
Jacksonville, Fla. 33617

Museum of Science and Industry
4801 East Fowler Avenue
Tampa, Fla. 33617

Museum of Science and Space Transit
Planetarium
3280 South Miami Avenue
Miami, Fla. 33129

Orlando Science Center*
810 East Rolling Street
Orlando, Fla. 32803-7151

Planet Ocean
3979 Rickenbacker Causeway
Miami, Fla. 33133

Science Museum and Planetarium of Palm
Beach County
4801 Dreher Trail
West Palm Beach, Fla. 33405

Space Coast Science Center
1510 Highland Avenue
P.O. Box 36-1816
Melbourne, Fla. 32936

Georgia

Fernbank Science Center*
156 Heaton Park Drive, N.E.
Atlanta, Ga. 30307

Georgia Southern Museum
Rosenwald Building, Box 8061
Georgia Southern College
Statesboro, Ga. 30460-8061

Hawaii

Bernice Pauahi Bishop Museum
P.O. Box 19000-A
1525 Bernice Street
Honolulu, Hawaii 96817-0916

Idaho

Idaho Museum of Natural History
Idaho State University
South 5th and Dillon
Pocatello, Idaho 83209

Illinois

Chicago Academy of Sciences
2001 North Clark Street
Chicago, Ill. 60614

Chicago Botanic Garden
P.O. Box 400
Glencoe, Ill. 60022

Discovery Center Museum
401 South Main Street
Rockford, Ill. 61101

Lakeview Museum of Arts and Sciences
1125 West Lake Avenue
Peoria, Ill. 61614

Museum of Science and Industry
57th Street and Lake Shore Drive
Chicago, Ill. 60637

Sci Tech*
18 W. Benton Street
Aurora, Ill. 60506

Indiana

The Children's Museum
P.O. Box 3000
Indianapolis, Ind. 46206

Evansville Museum of Arts and Sciences
411 S.E. Riverside Drive
Evansville, Ind. 47713

Indiana State Museum
202 North Alabama Street
Indianapolis, Ind. 46204

Iowa

Des Moines Center of Science and Industry
4500 Grand Avenue
Greenwood Park
Des Moines, Iowa 50312

Science Station*
427 First Street, S.E.
Cedar Rapids, Iowa 52401

The Children's Museum*
533 16th Street
Bettendorf, Iowa 52722

Kansas

Kansas Health Museum
3090 Main Street
Halstead, Kans. 67056

Museum of Natural History
University of Kansas
Lawrence, Kans. 66045

Kentucky

Museum of History and Science
727 West Main Street
Louisville, Ky. 40202

Louisiana

Louisiana Arts and Science Center*
P.O. Box 3373
Baton Rouge, La. 70821

Louisiana Children's Museum
New Orleans, La. 70130

Maryland

Maryland Science Center
Mary Hyman, Director, Education Department
601 Light Street
Baltimore, Md. 21230

Massachusetts

Children's Museum
Museum Wharf—300 Congress Street
Boston, Mass. 02210

The Computer Museum
300 Congress Street
Boston, Mass. 02210

Museum of Science
Science Park
Boston, Mass. 02114

Springfield Science Museum
236 State Street
Springfield, Mass. 01103

Worcester Science Center
222 Harrington Way
Worcester, Mass. 01604

Michigan

Alfred P. Sloan, Jr., Museum
1221 East Kearsley Street
Flint, Mich. 48503

Ann Arbor Hands-On Museum
219 East Huron Street
Ann Arbor, Mich. 41804

Cranbrook Institute of Science
500 Lone Pine Road
P.O. Box 801
Bloomfield Hills, Mich. 48013

Detroit Science Center
5020 John R Street
Detroit, Mich. 48202

Hall of Ideas of the Midland Center for the Arts, Inc.
1801 West St. Andrews Road
Midland, Mich. 48640

Impression 5 Science Museum
200 Museum Drive
Lansing, Mich. 48933

Kalamazoo Public Museum
315 South Rose Street
Kalamazoo, Mich. 49007

Minnesota

Mayo Medical Museum—Mayo Foundation
200 First Street, S.W.
Rochester, Minn. 55905

The Science Museum of Minnesota
30 East 10th Street
St. Paul, Minn. 55101

Mississippi

Mississippi Museum of Natural Science*
111 North Jefferson St.
Jackson, Miss. 39202

Missouri

The Kansas City Museum
3218 Gladstone Boulevard
Kansas City, Mo. 64123

Missouri Botanical Garden
P.O. Box 299
St. Louis, Mo. 63166

St. Louis Science Center*
5050 Oakland Avenue
St. Louis, Mo. 63110

Montana

Museum of the Rockies
South 7th and Kagy Boulevard
Bozeman, Mont. 59717

Nebraska

Omaha Children's Museum
551 South 18th
Omaha, Nebr. 68102

University of Nebraska State Museum
14th and U Streets
Lincoln, Nebr. 68588-0338

New Hampshire

Montshire Museum of Science
45 Lyme Road
Hanover, N.H. 03755

New Mexico

Bradbury Science Center
Los Alamos National Lab MS-B286
Los Alamos, N.Mex. 87545

National Atomic Museum
P.O. Box 5400
Kirtland Air Force Base
Albuquerque, N.Mex. 87115

The Space Center
P.O. Box 533
Alamogordo, N.Mex. 88311-0533

New York

The Brooklyn Children's Museum
145 Brooklyn Avenue
Brooklyn, N.Y. 11213

Buffalo Museum of Science
Humboldt Parkway
Buffalo, N.Y. 14211

The Discovery Center
321 South Clinton Street
Syracuse, N.Y. 13202

New York Hall of Science
47-01 111th Street
Corona, N.Y. 11368

Roberson Center for the Arts and Sciences
30 Front Street
Binghamton, N.Y. 13905

The Schenectady Museum and Planetarium
Nott Terrace Heights
Schenectady, N.Y. 12308

Science Discovery Center of Tomkins County
P.O. Box 6697
Ithaca, N.Y. 14851

Science Museum of Long Island
1526 North Plandome Road
Manhasset, N.Y. 11030

North Carolina

Catawba Science Center
234 3rd Avenue, N.E.
Hickory, N.C. 28601
Mailing Address:
P.O. Box 2431
Hickory, N.C. 27603

Health Adventure
501 Biltmore Avenue
Asheville, N.C. 28806

Natural Science Center
4301 Lawndale Drive
Greensboro, N.C. 27408

Nature Science Center
Museum Drive
Winston-Salem, N.C. 27105

North Carolina Museum of Life and Science
443 Murray Avenue
P.O. Box 15190
Durham, N.C. 57704

Schiele Museum of Natural History and Planetarium, Inc.
P.O. Box 953
1500 East Garrison Boulevard
Gastonia, N.C. 28053

Science Museums of Charlotte, Inc.
Beverly Sanford, Director of Education and Programs
Discovery Place and Charlotte Nature Museum
301 North Tryon Street
Charlotte, N.C. 28202

Ohio

Center of Science and Industry*
280 East Broad Street
Columbus, Ohio 43215

Cincinnati Museum of Natural History
1720 Gilbert Avenue
Cincinnati, Ohio 45202

Cleveland Children's Museum
11300 Juniper Road
Cleveland, Ohio 44106

Cleveland Health Education Museum
8911 Euclid Avenue
Cleveland, Ohio 44106

Museum of Health, Science, and Industry
Cincinnati Union Terminal
1301 Western Avenue
Cincinnati, Ohio 45203

NASA Lewis Research Center MS 8-1
Visitor Information Center
21000 Brookpark Road
Cleveland, Ohio 44135

Oklahoma

Omniplex
2100 N.E. 52nd Street
Oklahoma City, Okla. 73111

Oregon

Oregon Museum of Science and Industry*
4015 S.W. Canyon Drive
Portland, Oreg. 97221

Pennsylvania

Academy of Natural Sciences
19th Street and the Parkway
Philadelphia, Pa. 19103

Buhl Science Center
Allegheny Square
Pittsburgh, Pa. 15212

The Franklin Institute Science Museum*
20th Street and the Parkway
Philadelphia, Pa. 19103

Museum of Scientific Discovery
P.O. Box 934
Strawberry Square
Harrisburg, Pa. 17108

Reading Public Museum and Art Gallery
500 Museum Road
Reading, Pa. 19611-1425

South Carolina

Roper Mountain Science Center
504 Roper Mountain Road
Greenville, S.C. 29615-4229

Tennessee

American Museum of Science and Energy
300 South Tulane Avenue
Oak Ridge, Tenn. 37830

Cumberland Museum and Science Center
800 Ridley Boulevard
Nashville, Tenn. 37203-4899

Memphis Pink Palace Museum and Planetarium
3050 Central Avenue
Memphis, Tenn. 38111

Texas

Don Harrington Discovery Center
1200 Streit Drive
Amarillo, Tex. 79106

Fort Worth Museum of Science and History
1501 Montgomery Street
Forth Worth, Tex. 76107

Houston Museum of Natural Science*
1 Herman Circle Drive
Houston, Tex. 77030-1799

INSIGHTS—El Paso Science Center, Inc.
303 North Oregon
El Paso, Tex. 79901

McAllen International Museum
1900 Nolana
McAllen, Tex. 78504

The Petroleum Museum
Permian Basin Petroleum Museum, Library, and
Hall of Fame
1500 I-20 West
Midland, Tex. 79701

Science Place*
P.O. Box 151469
Fair Park
Dallas, Tex. 75315

Wichita Falls Museum and Art Center
Two Eureka Circle
Wichita Falls, Tex. 76302

Utah

Children's Museum of Utah
840 North 300 West
Salt Lake City, Utah 84103

Vermont

Vermont Institute of Natural Science
Church Hill
Woodstock, Vt. 05091

Virginia

Peninsula Nature and Science Center, Inc.
524 J. Clyde Morris Boulevard
Newport News, Va. 23601

The Roanoke Valley Science Museum Center
in the Square
One Market Square
Roanoke, Va. 24011

Science Museum of Virginia*
2500 West Broad Avenue
Richmond, Va. 23220

Virginia Museum of Transportation
802 Wiley Drive, S.W.
Roanoke, Va. 24015

Washington

Eastern Washington Science Center
Riverfront Park
North 507 Howard Street
Spokane, Wash. 99201
Mailing Address:
300 Patterson Hall
Eastern Washington University
Cheney, Wash. 99004

Hanford Science Center
P.O. Box 800
Richland, Wash. 99352

Pacific Science Center
Bill Schmitt, Director of Education
200 Second Avenue
Seattle, Wash. 98109

Wisconsin

Discovery World
Museum of Science, Economics, and Technology, Inc.
818 West Wisconsin Avenue
Milwaukee, Wis. 53233

Milwaukee Public Museum
800 West Wells Street
Milwaukee, Wis. 53233

Wyoming

High Plains Energy Technology Center*
P.O. Box 2500
Gillette, Wyo. 82717-2500

Magazines Dealing with Science and Technology

Current Science. Science articles geared toward youths of junior high school age. Field Publications, 245 Long Hill Road, Middletown, Conn. 06457.

National Geographic World. Science and travel articles for young people. Department 00887, 17th and M Streets, N.W., Washington, D.C. 20036.

Odyssey. Articles on space exploration and astronomy for young people. Kalmbach Publishing Company, 1027 North 7th Street, Milwaukee, Wis. 53233.

Ranger Rick Magazine. Articles on nature and wildlife for young people. National Wildlife Federation, 8925 Leesburg Pike, Vienna, Va. 22184-0001.

3-2-1 Contact. Articles on science and technology for young people. P.O. Box 53051, Boulder, Colo. 80322-2933.

Books That Encourage Exploration in Science and Technology

Note: Age levels for which books are best suited are denoted by D (Daisy), B (Brownie), J (Junior), C (Cadette), and S (Senior).

Abrusco, Joe, and Jack Hassard. *The Whole Cosmos Catalog of Science Activities.* Santa Monica, Calif.: Goodyear Publishing Company, 1977. A visually exciting and fun look at science, which includes activities, puzzles, games, and biographies of scientists. **(B, J, C)**

Allison, Linda. *Blood and Guts—A Working Guide to Your Own Insides.* Boston: Little, Brown and Company, 1976. Stories, experiments, and projects to introduce the reader to her own body. **(J, C)**

———. *The Reasons for Seasons: The Great Cosmic Megalactic Trip Without Moving from Your Chair.* Boston: Little, Brown and Company, 1975. Year-round science explorations. **(J, C)**

Bosak, Susan V. *Science Is . . .* A sourcebook of fascinating facts, projects and activities. Scholastic Canada LTD. Ontario, 1991. If you can get only one science book for working with kids, this is it! **(B, J, C, S, A)**

Burns, Marilyn. *The Book of Think, or How to Solve a Problem Twice Your Size.* Boston: Little, Brown and Company, 1976. Creative problem-solving, or "getting there from here." **(J, C)**

———. *Good for Me! All About Food in 32 Bites.* Boston: Little, Brown and Company, 1978. Explorations into foods, vitamins, good health, and the body. **(J, C)**

———. *The I Hate Mathematics Book.* Boston: Little, Brown and Company, 1975. Activities and fun approaches to math "magic," riddles, and problems. **(J, C)**

———. *Math for Smarty Pants.* Boston: Little, Brown and Company, 1982. Aspects of math for children and young people, with games and illustrations. **(J, C)**

———. *This Book Is About Time.* Boston: Little, Brown and Company, 1978. Activities about time, ranging from biological clocks to the making of timepieces. **(J, C)**

Carson, Mary Stetten. *The Scientific Kid.* Harper and Row Publishers, Inc. New York, 1989. Well illustrated activities for younger girls. **(D, B)**

Cobb, Vickie. *Science Experiments You Can Eat* (1972) and *More Science Experiments You Can Eat* (1979). New York: J. B. Lippincott Company. Excellent and fun introductions to scientific principles using the kitchen. Everything from chemistry to natural processes is included. **(B, J)**

Downey, Diane, Twila Slesnick, and Jean Stenmark. *Math for Girls and Other Problem Solvers.* Berkeley, Calif.: University of California, Lawrence Hall of Science, 1981. Contains fun strategy games that teach concepts in math and build problem-solving skills. **(B, J, C)**

Erickson, Tim. *Off and Running—The Computer OffLine Activities Book.* Berkeley, Calif.: EQUALS Project, Lawrence Hall of Science, 1986. Activities to introduce computer concepts and build computer literacy in a fun way. **(J, C)**

Fraser, Sherry. *Spaces: Solving Problems of Access to Careers in Engineering and Science.* Palo Alto, Calif.: EQUALS Project, Dale Seymour Publications, 1982. Fun activities designed to get young people thinking about scientific careers and to increase their interest in math. **(J, C)**

Hann, Judith. *How Science Works.* A Readers Digest book. Dorling Kindersley Ltd. London, 1991. A beautifully illustrated all-around science project book. **(B, J, C)** Other books in the Reader's Digest family science series include: *How Nature Works; How the Earth Works; and How the Universe Works.*

Kennedy, Carolyn. *Exploring Wildlife Communities with Children.* New York: Girl Scouts of the U.S.A., 1981. Hands-on learning about natural science in the out-of-doors. **(D, B, J, C, S)**

Lingelback, Jenepher. *Hands on Nature: Information and Activities for Exploring the Environment with Children.* Vermont Institute of Natural Science, Woodstock, Vt. 05091, 1987. Great outdoor investigations for children. Each activity has suggested readings. **(B, J)**

Outdoor Biological Instructional Strategies Program, Lawrence Hall of Science. *OBIS Activity Folders.* Delta Publishing, Box M, Nashua, N.H. 03061, 1981. Great hands-on environmental science activities for all ages. **(B, J, C, S)**

Rockwell, Robert E., Elizabeth A. Sherwood, and Robert A. Williams. *Hug a Tree and Other Things to Do Outdoors with Young Children.* Mt. Ranier, Md.: Gryphon House, 1983. Hands-on natural science activities for younger children. **(D, B)**

Ruef, Kerry. *The Private Eye. Looking/Thinking by Analogy. A Guide to Developing the Interdisciplinary Mind, Hands-on Thinking Skills, Creativity, Scientific Literacy.* The Private Eye Project, 7710 31st Ave. NW, Seattle, Wash. 98117, 1992. All you need is this book and a jeweler's loop to view the world differently! **(B, J, C, S)**

Stein, Sarah. *The Science Book.* New York: Workman Publishing, 1980. Has a fun format that encourages explorations in the world of science. **(J)**

Stenmark, Jean Kerr, Virginia Thompson, and Ruth Cossey. *Family Math.* Berkeley, Calif.: Lawrence Hall of Science, University of California, 1986. Focuses on parents and children learning math together through activities involving problem-solving skills and through hands-on activities. Available in Spanish edition as well. **(B, J, C)**

White, Lawrence B., Jr. *Science Games and Puzzles.* Reading, Mass.: Addison-Wesley, 1975. Interesting experiments for younger children that utilize materials found at home. **(D, B)**

Wyatt, Valerie. *The Science Book for Girls and Other Intelligent Beings.* Kids Can Press LTD, 1993. A delightful narrative with a different spin on "hands-on" science for girls. **(B, J, C)**

Other Resources

Square One TV Teachers' Guide. Children's Television Workshop, Box TG, One Lincoln Plaza, New York, N.Y. 10023. Price: $2.00 per copy; $1.00 per copy for 50 or more.

3-2-1 Contact Teachers' Guide (Sessions 2–6). Children's Television Workshop, Box TG, One Lincoln Plaza, New York, N.Y. 10023. Price: $5.00 per copy; $2.50 per copy for 50 or more.

Magic School Bus video series, (1994). Based upon Scholastic's book series of the same name, this PBS series is available through local PBS stations. Your council should have a copy of the teacher's guide. (Programs may be taped for educational purposes and used for three years.)

An Income of Her Own is an entrepreneurial network that offers girls and young women programs and materials for economic empowerment. Among the tools are: *Exploring Entrepreneurship Kit* (complete with game and leader's guide) which can be used to introduce girls and young women (ages 12-adult) to entrepreneurship and economic literacy so they can learn the language and ideas of business in fun and entertaining ways. Write or call AIOHO at P.O. Box 987, Santa Barbara, Calif. 93102 – (800) 350-2978 or (805) 646-1215 for more information about: The National Business Plan Competition for Teens (ages 13-18), Camp Enterprise, AIOHO Conferences/Video; AIOHO On-line, on becoming a member. Membership includes regular mailings, newsletters, and invitations to special events and much more!

The Stock Market Game (SMG), sponsored nationally by the Securities Industry Foundation for Economic Education, is a ten week simulation of stock market trading that provides a user-friendly framework for teaching youngsters about the American economic system. It can be used as a catalyst for further study of and interest in the American free enterprise system. For further information, contact the Securities Industry Foundation for Economic Education at (212) 608-1500.

Science-by-Mail

Museum of Science, Science Park, Boston, Mass. 02114-1099. Science packets with challenging activities that link girls with a scientist pen pal. Price: $56 per membership group of one to four kids. (Three packets in a membership year.) **(B, J, C)**

Women's History Catalog (yearly) available from National Women's History Project, 7738 Bell Road, Windsor, Calif. 95492-8518. Includes a wonderful collection of biographies, reference books, posters, and videos on women in science from past to present. Emphasis on multicultural contributions. Excellent resources for program centers and libraries, as well as special events.

Notes

Notes